YOUR KNOWLEDGE HAS VALUE

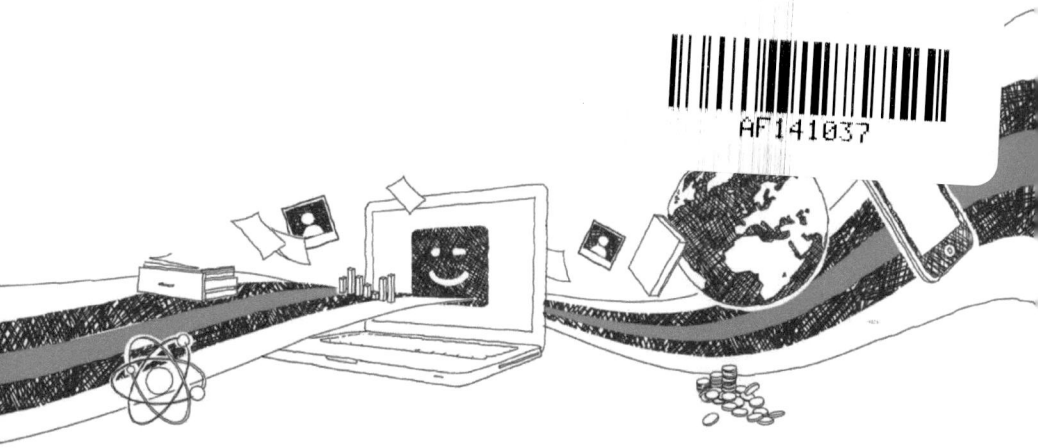
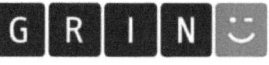

Prevalence of ovine and caprine babesiosis in Baligubadle-District. An empirical study

Ridwan Mohamed

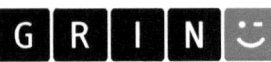

Bibliographic information published by the German National Library:

The German National Library lists this publication in the National Bibliography; detailed bibliographic data are available on the Internet at http://dnb.dnb.de.

ISBN: 9783346296931
This book is also available as an ebook.

© GRIN Publishing GmbH
Nymphenburger Straße 86
80636 München

Print and binding: Books on Demand GmbH, Norderstedt, Germany
Printed on acid-free paper from responsible sources.

The present work has been carefully prepared. Nevertheless, authors and publishers do not incur liability for the correctness of information, notes, links and advice as well as any printing errors.

GRIN web shop: https://www.grin.com/document/948233

PREVALENCE OF OVINE AND CAPRINE BABESIOSIS IN BALIGUBADLE DISTRICT, SOMALILAND

BY

RIDWAN OSMAN MOHAMED

THIS SPECIAL PROJECT WAS SUBMITTED IN PARTIAL FULFILLMENT OF THE REQUIREMENTS FOR THE AWARD OF DIPLOMA IN LIVESTOCK PRODUCT DEVELOPMENT AND ENTREPRENEURSHIP (DLDE) FROM IGAD SHEIKH TECHNICAL VETERINARY SCHOOL AND REFERENCE CENTRE, SOMALILAND.

JULY, 2015

DEDICATION

To my parents and whole family for their encouragement and love to me during my study and project writing.

ACKNOWLEDGEMENT

I would like to first thank to Allah the lord of the cosmos and the creator of features and appearances of the universe; who allow me to accomplish this mini-thesis in which none of this would have been possible without Allah for my Diploma graduate.

Secondly my family, specially my beloved parents to whom this thesis is dedicated my mother Fosia Hassan Omer and my father Osman Mohamed Sead with thier constant source of love, concern, assisting, generosity, understand, patience, leading, support and strength all these years. Eventually I would like to express my heart-felt, warmly appreciation and gratitude to my uncles Sulub Mohamed Sead, Abdihakim Hassan Omer and my brother Mukhtar Osman Mohamed, my two aunts Nim'o A/Rahman Yusouf and Awo A/Rahman Yusouf, my grandmothers and my grandfather, brothers, sisters, uncles, aunts, nephews and nieces to my all families to their positive attitude helping, to guide and support me during my study and Mini-thesis writing.

I am very thankful to my supervisor, Dr. Abdirahim Mohamed Garuum who has been an excellent mentor and guidance to me. I really appreciate the motivation, knowledge and support I received from him. I would also like to thank Tutor assistants Mousa and Nashad for their best time during my lab activity and positive consultant, and opportunity to final of my graduate mini-thesis.

All my friends have helped me to collect samples and data of this book through the difficult moment. Especially I would like to thank Mr. Kaisa Hassan and Ahmed Nour Osman their best support and care helped me overcome setbacks and stay focused on my graduate study. I greatly value their friendship and I deeply appreciate their confidence in me.

I am very grateful for all the technical assistance I received from lab technicians at diagnostic laboratory of Somaliland ministry of livestock, Hargeisa, who guided me through my first steps in the laboratory as well as the assistances of Yasir and Suhur Abdihakim.

Last but not least, I would like to acknowledge everyone in IGAD Sheikh Technical Veterinary School which includes tutors, graduate students, staff and all involvers.

TABLE OF CONTENTS

LIST OF FIGURES

ABBREVIATIONS

D	Margin of Error At 5% (Standard Value of 0.05)
DIC	Disseminated Intravascular Coagulation
EDTA	Ethylene Diamine Tetra-acetic Acid
ELISA	Enzyme-linked immunosorbent assay
Eng.	Example
i.e.,	That is To Say
IFAT	Inflorescence Antibody Test
ISTVS	IGAD Sheikh Technical Veterinary School
N	Required Sample Sizes
PEXP	Estimated Prevalence of Cattle with Ticks (50%)
T	Confidence Level At 95% (Standard Value of 1.96)
TBDs	Tick Borne Diseases
Yr	Year
GDP	Gross Domestic Product

ABSTRACT

Ovine and caprine babesiosis is an acute or chronic infectious disease of sheep and goats, caused by two species of Babesia, transmitted by ticks, and characterized by fever, anemia, hemoglobinuria and icterus. Ovine and caprine babesiosis is caused by two antigenically different species of Babesia: *B. motasi*, is a large and more virulent form, occurring singly or paired in erythrocytes; *B. ovis* which is a small form. The main objective of this study was to establish the prevalence of Babesiosis in sheep and goats in Baligubadle District, Somaliland.

Cross sectional study that has been carried out at 19 April up to 15 July in five villages in Baligubadle district. A total of 350 sheep and goats were sampled. Slides were made from a whole blood collected from the auricular vein of the animals. After staining, slides were read under a light microscope.

A prevalence of 3.4% of Babesiosis was found. The number of positives was more in young and sheep due to their weak immunity and less sensitiveness to ticks respectively.

The disease is locally known as *Kaadi dhiig* because of the characteristic red colored urine of the infected animals. Dipping and plants such as Gagabood are used to control ticks transmitting the disease.

Key Words: Prevalence, Ovine and Caprine Babesiosis, Sheep, Goat, Baligubadle. Somaliland

CHAPTER ONE: INTRODUCTION

1.1 Background Information

In sheep and goats, babesiosis is caused by B. ovis and B. motasi. Rhipicephalus bursa has been shown to be a vector for B. ovis while B. motasi is transmitted by ticks of the genus Haemaphysalis (*H. Punctata, H. Otophila*), Dermacentor (*D. silvarum*) and Rhipicephalus (*R. Bursa*) (Taylor *et al.*, 2007).

The babesias are one of the most ubiquitous and widespread blood parasites in the world based on numbers and distribution of species in animals, second only to the trypanosomes (Levine, N. D., 1988; Telford, S. R., et al, 1993). They generally have two classes of hosts, an invertebrate and a vertebrate host. The maintenance of *Babesia* spp. is dependent on both hosts; the specific tick vector must feed on a vertebrate reservoir that is competent in maintaining the *Babesia* organisms in an infectious state. Therefore, *B. microti* presents itself as an emerging zoonosis only in areas where there is a primary competent reservoir.

Babesiosis, caused by infection with intraerythrocytic parasites of the genus *Babesia*, is one of the most common infections of free-living animals worldwide and is gaining increasing interest as an emerging zoonosis in humans. Although capable of infecting a wide range of vertebrates, babesial parasites require both a competent vertebrate and non-vertebrate host to maintain transmission cycles. All babesial parasites described to date are transmitted by ixodid ticks to their vertebrate hosts. The parasites replicate in the vertebrate hosts' red blood cells and are called piroplasms due to their pear-shaped appearance when within the infected host cells (Kakoma, I., and H. Mehlhorn. 1993; Telford, S. R., et al, 1993). Most of what is known about the host response to babesial infections comes from observations of and studies on vertebrates other than humans. All mammalian hosts examined have been able to develop immunity to *Babesia* species, either after an episode of infection and recovery or after prophylactic immunization. Both humoral and cellular factors are involved in immunity to babesiosis.

Babesias can be found wherever certain species of ticks flourish. To date, only ixodid ticks have been identified as vectors for *Babesia* spp. except for one report that identified a nonixodes tick, *Ornithodoros erraticus*, as a reservoir for *Babesia meri* (Gunders, A. E., 1977).

2

Microscopic examinations revealed presence of Babesia parasites in sheep erythrocytes. PCR analysis confirmed the presence of 239 bp specific band corresponding to the DNA of Babesia species. Of the 395 sheep sampled, 22 (5.6%) were positive for Babesia spp. upon microscopic examination whereas 13 (3.3%) were positive for the presence of Babesia spp by PCR (Khansa, et al; 2017).

Economic losses result from deaths among affected sheep and goats, unthrifitiness of chronic cases, and the cost of control programs. Ovine and caprine babesiosis occurs in all breeds and sexes of sheep and goats, but animals 6-12 months old have a higher incidence than animals of other age groups (El Sawaly, A. A., 1999). Babesiosis, Theileriosis and Ehrelichiosis (Cowdriosis and Anaplasmosis) are the major TBDs that cause serious diseases among Central and East African animals including goats (E. J. L. Soulsby, 1986, A. M. El Hussein, et al., 2004).

Haemoprotozoan parasites are the main livestock production constraints all over the world (E. J. L. Soulsby, 1986., G. M. Urquhart, et al., 1996., K. T. Friedhoff, 1988). Causing serious economical losses; tick and tick borne diseases (T & TBDs) still remain to be a major threat to animals in tropical and sub tropical countries (E. J. L. Soulsby, 1986, A. M. El Hussein, et al., 2004, S. M. Hassan and D. A. Salih, 2009) including Somalia. In case of these blood parasites infection up to 75% erythrocytes may be destroyed in fatal cases and even in milder infection so many erythrocytes are destroyed, then a severe anaemia result (E. J. L. Soulsby, 1986; G. M. Urquhart, et al., 1996).

Research study conducted in Somalia, Benadir, samples were 22 samples (22%) were harboring single infection of Babesia spp. and 14 samples (14%) were having single infection of Theileria spp. Interestingly the Remaining 64 blood samples (64%) showed mixed infection of Babesia spp. with Theileria spp. were identified from the investigated goats Ahmed Abdulkadir *et al*, (2013).

This study was undertaken to know the Babesiosis prevalent in Ovine and Caprine in Baligubadle District, Hawd region, Somaliland. This study will add an additional advantage of the Babesiosis cover the further pave the way for launching sustainable animal disease controlling and minimizing in Somaliland.

However there is little data on national herd distribution and composition up to date. Furthermore there is little information about the prevalence of Babesiosis in sheep and goats in Baligubadle district, therefore this study is aimed at investigating the prevalence of sheep and goats Babesiosis in Baligubadle district, Somaliland.

1.2 Problem Statement

Somaliland has 14.3 million herds of Sheep and Goats, 1.5 million herds of Camel and about 0.4 million herds of cattle (National livestock policy, 2006) and about 60% of the economy of Somaliland depends on livestock. Besides the local consumption, Sheep and Goats are the major livestock species exported to generate currency.

Due to the poor veterinary infrastructure, the uncontrolled use of drugs and the abundance of ticks; Sheep and Goats are susceptible to tickborne diseases including babesiosis.

In addition the free movement of sheep and goats across the border of Somaliland and Ethiopia makes sheep and goat more susceptible to Babesiosis.

Furthermore, there are no much awareness about the impacts of Babesiosis on sheep and goats and there is limited data about the prevalence of Sheep and Goat Babesiosis. Therefore this study is aimed at assessing the prevalence of Sheep and Goat Babesiosis in Baligubande district, Somaliland.

1.3 justification and significance of the study

Sheep and goat Babesiosis is production-limiting disease and due to the poor veterinary service, the uncontrolled veterinary drug used and the abundance of ticks, sheep and goats are at risk getting Babesiosis. Due to the high number of livestock, owners does not give a continuous disease check up for their livestock thus the disease is poorly controlled and there is poor understanding the impacts and the magnitude of the disease. In addition, there is limited information about Babesiosis in Sheep and Goats in Somaliland,

Therefore this study will establish the prevalence of Babesiosis in sheep and goats in Baligubadle district, Somaliland.

The results from this study are expected to be used by the ministry of livestock and other local and international NGOs to address Babesiosis in and the predisposing factors in sheep and goats.

1.4 Objectives

1.4.1 General Objectives

The main objective of this study is to establish the prevalence of Babesiosis in sheep and goats in Baligubadle District, Somaliland.

1.4.2 Specific Objectives

1. To determine the prevalence of ovine and caprine Babesiosis in Baligubadle district in sheep and goats.

2. To compare the prevalences of age and species of sheep and goats Babesiosis.

3. To determine the indigenous knowledge about the prevention Ovine and Caprine Babesiosis

CHAPTER TWO: LITERATURE REVIEW

2.1 Background of Babesiosis

Ovine and caprine babesiosis is an acute or chronic infectious disease of sheep and goats, caused by two species of Babesia, transmitted by ticks, and characterized by fever, anemia, hemoglobinuria and icterus. Ovine and caprine babesiosis is caused by two antigenically different species of Babesia: B. motasi, is a large and more virulent form, occurring singly or paired in erythrocytes; B. ovis, is a small form. Ovine and caprine babesiosis is widespread in tropical and subtropical regions as North Africa including Egypt, the Middle East, southeastern Europe, and South America. Ticks of the genera Dermacentor, Rhipicephalus, Haemaphysalis, and Ixodes have been incriminated as vectors. The organisms are transmitted transovarially or transstadially depending on the vector involved. Intrauterine transmission of B. ovis also occurs. Ovine and caprine babesiosis occurs in all breeds and sexes of sheep and goats, but animals 6-12 months old have a higher incidence than animals of other age groups. The disease has a seasonal occurrence (El Sawaly, A. A., 1999).

2.2 Etiology

Babesiosis is a parasitic infection due to the multiplication of *Babesia* sp. in erythrocytes (Levine, 1985; Piesman, 1987). Although small ruminants can be infected by several species of *Babesia*, the two most important species are *B ovis* and *B motasi*, transmitted by *Rhipicephalus bursa* and *Haemaphysalis* spp, respectively (Phillip D. Carter; 2015). Genus *Babesia* consists of group of intracellular parasites with around hundred species (Uilenberg, 2001; Yakhchali & Hossein 2006).

2.3 Lifecycle of the Tick

Rhipicephalus. Bursa is two-host tick that occurs from the Mediterranean Basin down to the Middle East. It prefers mild climates, neither too cool, nor to hot. It attacks sheep and goats, as well as many wild species. Engorged adult females measured up to 1 cm in length. Larvae attach to hosts in autumn and molt to nymphs till deep in the winter. They drop off to the ground and molt to adults, which become active in spring and remain infective through the whole summer. The life cycle takes about 9 months. *Rhipicephalus bursa* can transmit numerous microbial diseases of livestock such as various species of *Babesia* leading those cause ovine and caprine babesiosis *B. ovis and B, motasi* (Phillip D. Carter and Peter Rolls, 2015) and (Taylor *et al.*, 2007).

6

2.4 Epidemiology

Although small ruminants can be infected by several species of *Babesia*, the two most important species are *B ovis* and *B motasi*, transmitted by *Rhipicephalus bursa* and *Haemaphysalis* spp, respectively. Infection is of importance in the Middle East, southern Europe, and some African and Asian countries (Phillip D. Carter and Peter Rolls, 2015).

In endemic areas, three features are important in determining the risk of clinical disease: firstly kids and lambs have a degree of immunity (related both to colostral-derived antibodies and to age-specific factors) that persists for ~6 month of age, secondly animals that recover from *Babesia* infections are generally immune for their commercial life (4 yr), and thirdly the susceptibility of sheep and goats breeds to ticks and *Babesia* infections varies, while other tend to be more resistant to ticks and the effects of *B ovis* and *B motasi* infection (Phillip D. Carter and Peter Rolls, 2015).

At high levels of tick transmission, virtually all lambs and kids become infected with *Babesia* by 6 moth of age, show few if any clinical signs, and subsequently become immune. This situation can be upset by either a natural (eg, climatic) or artificial (eg, acaricide treatment or changing breed composition of herd) reduction in tick numbers to levels such that tick transmission of *Babesia* to sheep and goats is insufficient to ensure all are infected during this critical early period. Strain variation in immunity has been demonstrated but is probably not of practical significance in the field (Phillip D. Carter and Peter Rolls, 2015).

2.4.1 Transmission

The transmission of Babesia parasites is mostly through the bite of infected ticks during blood sucking. The merozoites are introduced; they invade host erythrocytes, reproduce asexually and form a pair of trophozoites. The trophozoites are released. They re-invade other red blood cells and lead to intravascular haemolysis and anaemia. Iatrogenic transmission with repeated use of hypodermic needle without sterilization in hospitals or during mass vaccination may also take place. The main consequence of the disease was haemolytic anaemia (Habibi et al., 2004; Sevinc et al., 2007) results from mechanical damage (Callow and Pepper, 1974), autoimmune phenomena (Argon, 1976), increased host erythrocyte permeability (Alkhalil et al., 2007) and erythrophagocytosis by activated macrophage (Saleh, 2009). The parasite is transmitted by ticks of

7

the genus Haemaphysalis (H. Punctata, H. Otophila), Dermacentor (D. silvarum) and Rhipicephalus (R. Bursa) (Taylor *et al.*, 2007).

2.4.2. Disease Geographical Distribution

Ovine and caprine babesiosis is widespread in tropical and subtropical regions as North Africa including Egypt, the Middle East, southeastern Europe, and South America (El Sawaly, A. A., 1999).

2.4.3 Host Range

Ovine nad caprine babesiosi occurs in all breeds and sexes of sheep and goats, but animals 6-12 months old have a higher incidence than animals of other age groups. The disease has a seasonal occurrence (El Sawaly, A. A., 1999).

2.5 Pathogenesis

Babesia produces acute disease by two principle mechanism; hemolysis and circulatory disturbance (Carlton WW and MD Mc Gavin, 1995). During the tick bite, sporozoites are injected into the host and directly infect red blood cells. In the host, Babesia sporozoites develop into piroplasms inside the infected erythrocyte resulting in two or sometimes four daughter cells that leave the host cell to infect other erythrocytes (Hunfeld KP, et al., 2008).

It invades erythrocyte and cause intravascular and extravascular hemolysis (Carlton WW and MD Mc Gavin, 1995). The rapidly dividing parasites in the red cells produce rapid destruction of the erythrocytes with accompanying haemoglobinaemia, haemoglobinuria and fever. This may be so acute as to cause death within a few days, during which the packed cell volume falls below 20% which will lead to anemia. The parasitaemia, which is usually detectable once the clinical signs appear, may involve between 0.2% up to 45% of the red cells, depending on the species of Babesia (Urquhart GM, et al., 1996).

Cytokines and other pharmacologically active agents have an important function in the immune response to Babesia. The outcome is related to the timing and quantity produced, but their overproduction contributes to disease progress causing vasodilation, hypotension, increased capillary permeability, oedema, vascular collapse, coagulation disorders, endothelial damage and circulatory stasis (Ahmed JS., 2002).

8

Although stasis is induced in the microcirculation by aggregation of infected erythrocytes in capillary beds, probably the most deleterious pathophysiological lesions occur in the brain and lung. This can result in cerebral babesiosis and a respiratory distress syndrome associated with infiltration of neutrophils, vascular permeability and oedema. Progressive haemolyticanaemia develops during the course of *B. bovis* infections. While this is not a major factor during the acute phase of the disease, it will contribute to the disease process in more protracted cases (Brown W C and Palmer GH., 1999).

B. bovis is the most pathogenic of the bovine Babesia. B. bigemina infections are not as virulent as those of B. bovis, however the parasites may infect 40% of the red cells (Taylor *et al.*, 2007). Babesia affecting small ruminants are generally less pathogenic than their bovine counterparts (Cebra, C., and Cebra, M., 2002).

2.6 Clinical Signs

In acute cases, affected sheep show fever, anemia, hemoglobinuria, icterus and weakness, and 30-40 % of affected sheep usually die. Chronically infected sheep usually are asymptomatic, except for parasitemia and unthriftiness (EI Sawaly, A. A., 1999).

2.7 Diagnosis

Diagnosis depends on the clinical signs and demonstration of Babesia species in blood smears. In case of sudden death, the disease should be differentiated from anthrax (EI Sawaly, A. A., 1999).

2.7.1 Clinical Diagnosis

Clinical manifestations of disease associated with BB are typical of a haemolytic anaemia disease process but vary according to agent (i.e. species of parasite) and host factors (i.e. age, immune status) (OIE Reference Laboratories for Bovine babesiosis, 2010).

2.7.2 Differential Diagnosis

Several diseases can be misdiagnostic with ovine and caprine babesiosis such as Anaplasmosis, Theileriosis, Bacillary haemoglobinuria, Leptospirosis, Eperythrozoonosis, Rapeseed poisoning and Chronic copper poisoning are one of diseases require not to under mistake this disease (OIE Reference Laboratories for Bovine babesiosis, 2010).

2.8 Laboratory Diagnosis

2.8.1 Sampling

Several thick and thin blood smears collected from superficial skin capillaries (e.g. tip of the ear or tip of the tail) of live animals during the acute phase of the disease (appearance of fever). Thin blood films should be air-dried, fixed in absolute methanol for 1 minute and stained with 10% Giemsa stain for 20–30 minutes. Blood films should be stained as soon as possible after preparation to ensure proper stain definition. Thick films are made by placing a small drop (approximately 50 µl) of blood on to a clean glass slide and spreading this over a small area using a circular motion with the corner of another slide. The droplet is air-dried, heat-fixed at 80°C for 5 minutes, and stained (without fixing in methanol) in 10% Giemsa for 15 minutes. Unstained blood films should not be stored with or near formalin solutions as formalin fumes may affect staining quality; moisture also affects staining quality. If it is not possible to make fresh films from capillary blood, sterile jugular blood should be collected into an anticoagulant such as lithium heparin or ethylene diamine tetra-acetic acid (EDTA) (Invasive Species Compendium; 2015).

2.8.1.1 Procedures of Sampling Testing

Identification of the agent

Microscopic examination of blood the traditional method of identifying agents in infected animals by microscopic examination of Giemsa-stained thick and thin blood films

- Stained films are examined under oil immersion using (as a minimum) a ×8 eyepiece and a ×60 objective lens
- Morphology of *Babesia* described in various sources,

10

- Sensitivity of thick films can detect parasitaemias as low as 1 parasite in 106 red blood cells
- *Babesia* species differentiation is good in thin films but poor in the more sensitive thick films
- Adequate for detection of acute infections, but not for detection of carriers where parasitaemias are very low
- Parasite identification and differentiation improved by using a fluorescent dye, such as acridine orange instead of Giemsa (Invasive Species Compendium; 2015).

2.9 Treatment and Control

After the hemoglobinuria or cerebral signs, prognosis is not good. In acute cases that PVC values are above 12%, treatment will be successful. Supportive therapy such as blood transfusions (4 L of whole blood per 250 kg of body weight), fluids, hematinics, and prophylactic antibiotics are important (Zaugg, 2009).

Babesiosis can be treated by using suh as diminazene aceturate (3-5 mg/ kg), phenemidine diisethionate (8-13 mg/ kg), imidocarb dipropionate (1-3 mg/kg), and amicarbalide diisethionate (5-10 mg /kg) (Cebra, C., and Cebra, M., 2002a; Taylor, 2007; Radostits, 2008; Zaugg, 2009). The control of the disease depends on effective quarantine to prevent the introduction of the vector tick. The control of ticks by dipping or spraying animals at risk with recommended acaricides. In routine surgery, care should be taken to prevent accidental transfer of blood from one animal to another (e.g., castration, dehorning). In addition, in cattle, the selection and breeding of cattle which acquire a high degree of resistance to ticks is practiced. Widespread use of tick vaccines may also have a significant influence on the incidence of infection in cattle (Taylor *et al.*, 2007; Radostits *et al.*, 2008; Zaugg, 2009).

CHAPTER THREE: METHODOLOGY

3.1 Study Area

Baligubadle District is 62 km south of Hargeisa; the district serves as the capital of Hawd Region. An administration was established by Somaliland and was created in 2008. It has boundaries with Maroodi-Jeeh Region in the north, Daad-Madheedh Region in the east, Gabiley Region in the west and Ethiopia in the south. According to the office of the Mayor, the district has a population of 50,000 and administers over 34 communities or villages including: Gumarta, Bidhiiqa, Bali Case, Kaabada Bari, Warta Mohamed Farah, Ina Cunaaye, Darafacle, Habaasweyne, Jabaaqa, Dhiishka, Magaalo Haalay, Hunguri-Gorayo, Gumburaha, and kaabada Galbeed. This district boeder line district while tick borne diseases has a higher comlain to the community. While thier animals are market oriented and animals are always transport in and out Somaliland and Ethiopia.

3.2 Study Design

Cross-sectional study design was implemented to determine the prevalence of sheep and goat Babesiosis in Baligubadle District. A total of 350 sheep and goats were sampled from five randomly selected villages. Study animals were divided in to two strata (sheep and goats) and each stratum was selected using simple random sampling.

3.3 Study Population

The study population consisted of randomly selected 350 sheep and goats in Baligubadle district which were kept under traditional extensive systems.

3.4 Sample Size

According to Thrusfield, (1995), the sample size was determined by using a 95% CI, 5% precision and with an expected prevalence of 50% (No previous prevalence).

$$n= \frac{t^2 \times pexp(1-pexp)}{d^2}$$

Where

n = required sample sizes

t = confidence level at 95% (standard value of 1.96)

pexp = estimated prevalence of cattle with ticks (50%)

d = margin of error at 5% (standard value of 0.05)

Therefore, $(1.96)^2 * 0.5(1-0.5)/ (0.05)^2$

385 of sheep and goats however due to time and finincial constraints, **350** sheep and goat were sampled.

3.5 Sampling Method

Villages were selected using simple random sampling while animals were sampled using stratified sampling, the animals was first divided in to two strata (sheep and goats), then sheep and goats was randomly sampled from each strata to get a representative sample of Sheep and Goats.

Blood samples were collected from the auricular vein of the animals. Thin blood smears were made and fixed with 70% ethanol for ten seconds. Then the slide were stained with Giemsa stain and examined under the microscope at X100 objective (oil immersion objective) to detect Babesia parasite.

Questionnaires were used to identify the awareness of the disease, economic impacts and prevention and control methods of Babesiosis in Goats and Sheep.

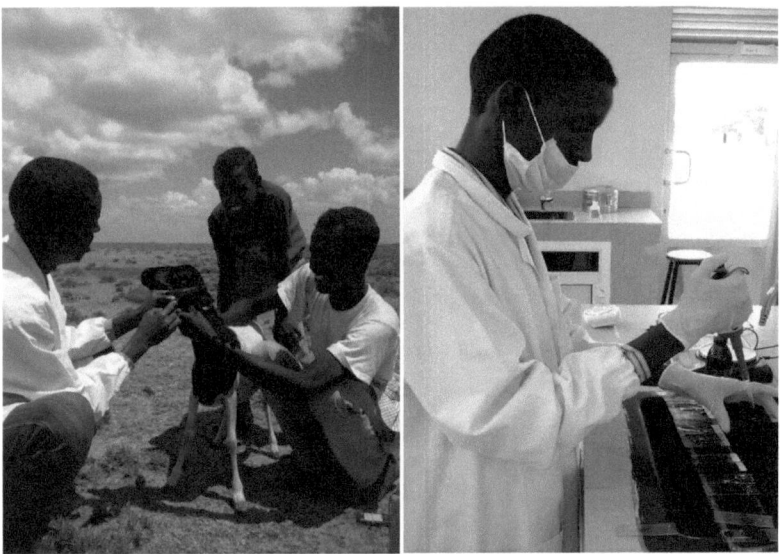

Figure 1: Bleeding a sheep - own work   **Figure 2: Staining blood smears - own work**

3.6 Materials

Vacutainers with EDTA, syringes and needles, slides, oil immersion, geimsa stain, absolute alcohol, microscope, note book and pen, digital camera, marker, precaution clothes (coverall and gloves) and drugs.

3.7 Data Analysis

The collected data was analyzed using excel statistical package and the results were presented as tables, graphs and charts.

CHAPTER FOUR: RESULTS

A cross sectional study was carried out from 19 April up to 19 July 2015 to establish the prevalence of sheep and goats Babesiosis in Baligubadle district. A total of 350 sheep and goats were sampled from five randomly selected villages.

4.1 Democratic Characteristics of the Study Participants

Questionnaires were administered to ten selected sheep and goat owners in Baligubadle district it has been noticed that all the ten sheep and goat owners which were men and women have no informal education. The questionnaires were noticed that an information about the community awareness, economical impact and traditional treatments and prevention of sheep and goat Babesiosis in Baligubadle district.

4.2 Overall prevalence of Babesiosis

Out of the 350 animals sampled, 12 animals were positive with a prevalence of 3.4%.

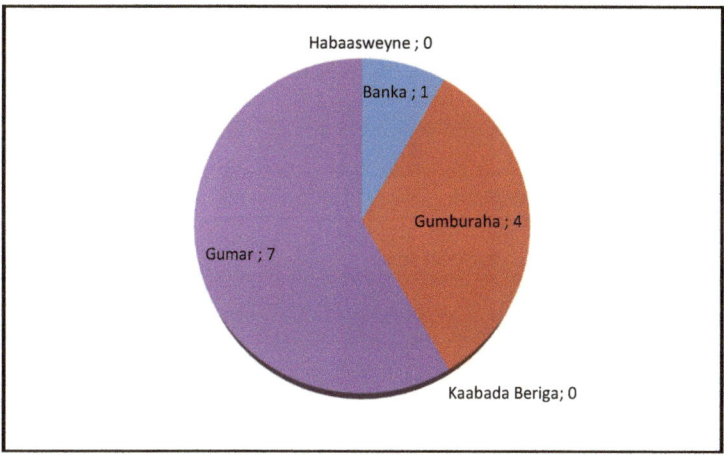

Figure 3: overall prevalence of Babesiosis

The pie chart above shows the prevalence of Babesiosis in study area with a percentage expression in each village, as shown the two villages of Kaabada Beriga and Habaasweyne have no a positive results after laboratory examination and shown zero result with no color have by them.

4.3 Prevalences of Babesiosis in Sheep and Goats

Prevalence in between sheep and goats of the study area has been a different number of cases positive which as shown Figure 2 as below follows.

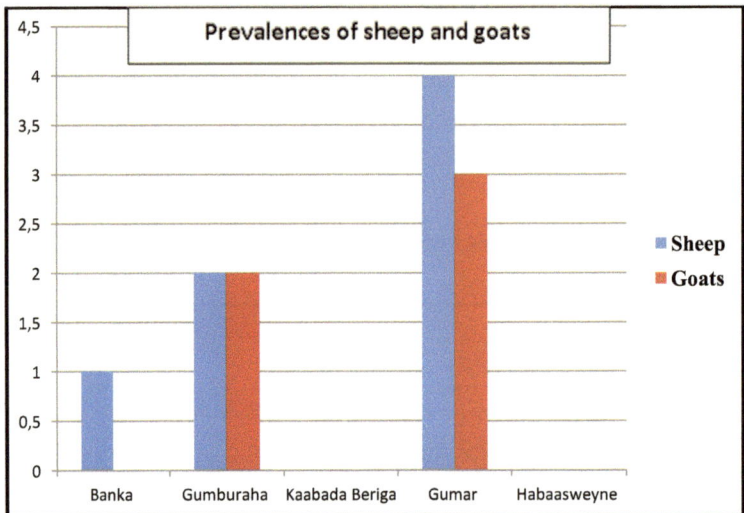

Figure 4: Prevalences of Babesiosis in sheep and goats

The figure above shows the prevalences of sheep and goats Babesiosis. According to the study, sheep had more positives than goats.

4.4 Prevalence of Babesiosis in Adult and Young of Sheep and Goats

Comparison of the prevalence of Babesiosis for young and adult sheep and goats were made according to the following graph.

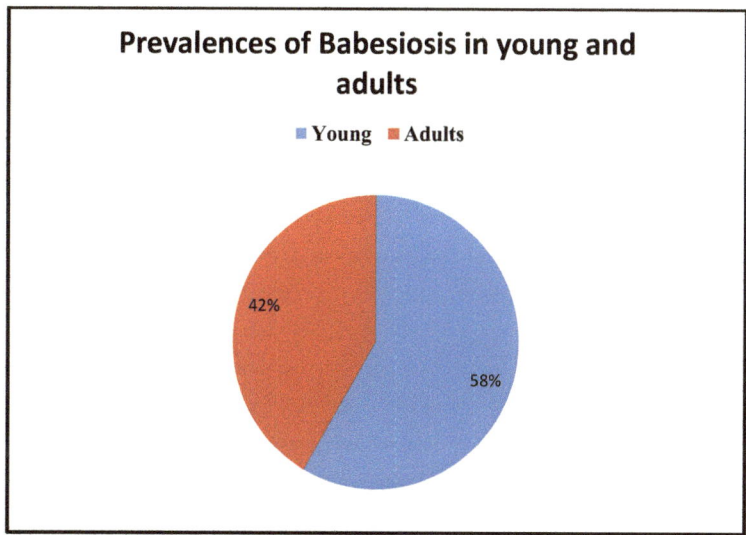

Figure 5: Prevalences for Babesiosis for adult and young sheep and goats

This percentage pie chart compares the prevalences of Babesiosis for young and adult sheep and goats in Baligubadle district. According to the graph, Babesiosis was higher in young animals compared to adult sheep and goats.

4.5 Traditional Knowledge about Sheep and Goat Babesiosis

Traditionally, Babesiosis is known as *Kaadi dhiig*. Dhoobley (*R. Bursa*) and Shilin cas (R. *evertsi*) was believed to be the vector of Babesiosis for sheep and goats. Anemia, anorexia, emaciation, loss of milk and meat production, abortion in rare cases and death in young animals. The control of the vector is achieved by controlling the vectors. Vectors are controlled by avoiding in highly infested areas and using some plants such as *Gagabood*.

CHAPTER FIVE: DISCUSSION

This study establishes the prevalence of sheep and goats in Baligubadle district. A prevalence of 3.4% was found. A study carried out by A. A. Hassan et al., (2013) reported a prevalence rate of 22% in Benadir region of Somalia. The differences of the prevalences to could be due different environments. Whereas the sun is hot in Baligubade district, Benadir region is climatically thought to favour ticks which transmit Babesiosis.

This study establishes the prevalences of sheep and goats Babesiosis. According to the study, sheep had more positives than goats when we compare the prevelances of sheep and goats Babesiosis. Which are 7 samples of positive in sheep of 58.33% compared to the goats of 5 positive samples 41.66%. Similar study carried out by (Iqbal F; et al, 2011) from Southern Punjab indicate similar prevalence compared the study results of revealed that 36 out of 107 sampled sheep and goats were positive for Babesia sp. 20 sheep and 16 goat blood samples were parasite positive. In that study, among 107 sampled animals 36 (34 %) were positive for Babesia sp., which shows the high prevalence of sheep in which 40 samples 20 of them become positive which is 50% of the total samples, while goats were 67 samples whereas 16 samples got positive result which is 24% from the total goat samples. this parasite in southern districts of Punjab.

The study established a relationship of the age of sheep and goats and Babesia infections. The study revealed a higher prevalence of Babesia infections in young sheep and goats (less than twelve months) compared to the adults. A study carried out by (EI Sawaly, A. A., 1999) at Egypt shows higher prevalences of Babesia infections in young sheep and goats. Young sheep and goats are more susceptible since their passive immune from their dams goes out and their immune still not well developed, they become susceptible as that. Adult animals have been exposure to those pathogens so many times and have developed their immune.

This study established livestock owners traditionally identified the disease with the red colored urine due to the destroyed red blood cells which are excreted in the urine and controlled the vector with some plant. Livestock owners controlled Babesia infection by controlling the vector controlling by hand removing technique, dipping and some traditional plants. This study is similar with the study of Piesman, J., et al, 1987 and Piesman, J., and A. Spielman. 1980 that indicate

18

preventive measures range from simple avoidance to habitat modification. Simple measures include use of tick repellents before entering a tick-infested area, avoidance of or minimization of exposure to tick-infested areas, and thorough examination of skin after exposure. Ticks found before attachment should obviously be removed, and ticks found after attachment can also be removed to limit the possibility of transmission if they can be removed within 24 h after attachment. Whereas Mather, T. N., et al; 1987 and Stafford, K. C., 3rd. 1991 carried out similar studies indicate the various public health measures have been put into effect which depend on reducing the density of the tick population. The use of acaricides is the most common method; the application of this pesticide to host nests and on the coats of reservoir hosts can interrupt transmission of *B. microti.*

CHAPTER SIX: CONCLUSIONS AND RECOMMENDATIONS

6.1 Conclusion

1. This study establishes the presence of Babesiosis in Somaliland. Prevalence of Babesiosis in sheep and goats in Baligubadle district is 3.4%.

2. Sheep had more positives than goats; the reason could be for the fact that sheep are less sensitive to ticks and thus are highly infested with ticks compared to goats.

3. Young animals had more positives than adult sheep and goats, this is because young sheep and goats have lower immune system compared to adult sheep and goats

4. The disease is locally known as *Kaadi dhiig* because of the characteristic red colored urine of the infected animals. Dipping and plants such as Gagabood are used to control ticks transmitting the disease.

6.2 Recommendation

- Due to the continuous movement of livestock across the borders of Somaliland it is possible that animals come with the disease or infected vectors in to Somaliland thus there is a need for control and inspect of animals before interring the borders of Somaliland,

- Livestock owners should be trained on the background, transmission, treatment and control of the disease.

- Continuous epidemiological surveillance is necessary for the treatment and control of the disease.

- Livestock owners should be taught on how to dip and use acaricides properly.

REFERENCES

1. A. M. El Hussein, A. M. Majid and S. M. Hassan, "The Present Status of Tick-Borne Diseases in the Sudan," Archives de l'Institut Pasteur de Tunis, Vol. 81, No. 5, 2004, pp. 31-34.

2. A. M. El Hussein, A. M. Majid and S. M. Hassan, "The Present Status of Tick-Borne Diseases in the Sudan," *Ar- chives de l'Institut Pasteur de Tunis*, Vol. 81, No. 5, 2004, pp. 31-34.

3. Abdalla, M., Ahmed, A. & Hamisi, S. (2017). Microscopic and Molecular Detection of Camel Anaplasmosis and Piroplasmosis in Banadir region, Somalia. *Open Access Journal of Veterinary Science & Research* 2(1): 2-8.

4. Ahlam F. Hamoda, *et al*; 2014; "Toxic Effect of Babesiosis in Cattle and Chemotherapiotic Treatment in Egypt." *American Journal of Infectious Diseases and Microbiology*, vol. 2, no. 5; Pg 91-96

5. Ahme d, Sadia M.; Ali, Hassan M.; and Wa same, Amina M. " Report on Research Finding on the

6. Ahmed Abdulkadir Hassan1, Abdalla Mohamed Ibrahim2, Rabab Haroon Mohamed and Hussein Haji Aden; 2013. Preliminary Assessment of Goat Piroplasmosis in Banadir Region, Somalia, *Open Journal of Veterinary Medicine*, 2013, 3, 273-276

7. Ahmed JS. The Role of Cytokines in Immunity and Immunopathogenesis of Pirolasmoses. Parasitol Res. 2002; 88: 48–50.

8. Alkhalil, A., Hill, D.A. and Desai, S.A. 2007. Babesia and plasmodia increase host erythrocyte permeability through distinct mechanisms. Cell Microbiol., 94: 815-860.

9. Armstrong, P. M., P. Katavolos, D. A. Caporale, R. P. Smith, A. Spielman, and S. R. Telford III. 1998. Diversity of *Babesia* infecting deer ticks (*Ixodes dammini*). Am. J. Trop. Med. Hyg. 58:739–742.

10. Brown W C, Palmer GH. Designing blood-stage vaccines against Babesiabovis and B. bigemina. Parasitol Today. 1999; 15: 275–281.

11. Brown WC, *et al*; 2006; Prospects for recombinant vaccines against *Babesia bovis* and related parasites. *Parasite Immunol.* ; pg 27-315.

12. Callow, L.L. and Pepper, P.R. 1974. Measurement and correlation between fever, changes in the packed cell volume and parasitemia in the evaluation of the susceptibility of cattle to infection with Babesia argentina. Aust. Vet J., 50:1-5.

13. Carlton WW, MD Mc Gavin. Thomson's Special Veterinary Pathology. 2nd ed. USA: Mosby Year Book Incorparted. 1995; 292-294.

14. Cebra, C., and Cebra, M., 2002a. Diseases of the Hematologic, Immunologic, and Lymphatic Systems (Multisystem Diseases). In: Pugh, D.G. (Eds): Sheep and Goat Medicine. Saunders, An Imprint of Elsevier. Philadelphia, Pennsylvania.

15. Cebra, C., and Cebra, M., 2002b. Diseases of the Cardiovascular System. In: Pugh, D.G. (Eds): Sheep and Goat Medicine. Saunders, An Imprint of Elsevier. Philadelphia, Pennsylvania.

16. Criado-Fornelio   A.   A;   2007;   review   of   nucleic-acid-based   diagnostic   tests for *Babesia* and *Theileria*, with emphasis on bovine piroplasms. *Parassitologia* : pg 39-44.

17. DELGADO, C., ROSEGRANT , M., STEINFELD, H ., EHUI , S. & COURBOIS, C. (1999). Livestock to 2020 : the next food revolution. Nairobi, Kenya, IFPRI/FAO/ILRI.
18. DELGADO, C., ROSEGRANT , M., STEINFELD, H ., EHUI , S. & COURBOIS, C. (1999). Livestock to 2020 : the next food revolution. Nairobi, Kenya, IFPRI/FAO/ILRI.
19. E. J. L. Soulsby, "Helminths, Arthropods & Protozoa of Domesticated Animals," 7th Edition, Bailliere Tindall, London, 1986.
20. El Sawalhy, A. A. (1999); "veterinary infectious diseases" 2nd Edition. Ovine and caprine babesiosis; *Ahram Distribution Agency*, Egypt. page 1
21. G. M. Urquhart, J. Armour, J. L. Duncan, A. M. Dunn and F. W. Jennings, "Veterinary Parasitology," 2nd Edition, B-Blackwell Science, 1996.
22. Gunders, A. E. 1977. Piroplasmal sporozoites in the argasid *Ornithodoros erraticus* (Lucas). Experientia 33:892–893.
23. Habibi, G.R., Hashemi-Fesharki, R., Bordbar, N. 2004. Detection of Babesia ovis using polymerase chain reaction. Arch. Razi Ins., 57: 1-10.
24. HASHEMI-FESHARKI R. Tick-borne diseases of sheep and goats and their related vectors in Iran. *Parasitology*, 1997, *39*, 115-117.
25. Hashemi-Fesharki R; 1997; Tick-borne diseases of sheep and goats and their related vectors in Iran. *Parassitologia*. pg 7-115.
26. Hunfeld KP, A Hildebrandt, JS Gray. Recent insights into Babesiosis. International Journal for Parasitology. 2008; 38: 1219-1237.
27. Invasive Species Compendium; 2015; Babesiosis; *overview of Babesiosis; data sheet of cookies invasive species compendium*; page 4 -5.
28. Invasive Species Compendium; 2015; Babesiosis; *overview of Babesiosis; data sheet of cookies invasive species compendium; page 4 -5.*
29. Iqbal F., Fatima M., Shahnawaz S., Naeem M., Shaikh R.S., Ali M., Shaikh A.S., Aktas M. And Ali M.; 2011; A study on the determination of risk factors associated with babesiosis and prevalence of babesia Sp., by PCR amplification, in small ruminants from Southern Punjab (Pakistan); *Parasite*, 2011, *18*, 229-234.
30. K. T. Friedhoff, "Transmission of Babesia," In: M. Ristic, Ed., Babesiosis of Domestic Animals and Man, CRC Press, Boca Raton, 1988, pp. 23-52.
31. Kakoma, I., and H. Mehlhorn. 1993. *Babesia* of domestic animals, p. 141– 216. *In* J. P. Kreier (ed.), Parasitic protozoa, 2nd ed., vol. 7. Academic Press, San Diego, Calif.
32. Levine N.D. Veterinary Protozoology. Iowa State University Press, Ames, 1985, 24-41.
33. Levine, N. D. 1988. The protozoan phylum apicomplexa, vol. 2. CRC Press, Boca Raton, Fla.
34. Mather, T. N., J. M. Ribeiro, and A. Spielman. 1987. Lyme disease and babesiosis: acaricide focused on potentially infected ticks. Am. J. Trop. Med. Hyg. 36:609–614.
35. OIE Reference Laboratories for Bovine babesiosis; (2010); *Bovine Babesiosis; diagnostic techniques*; page 2-7.
36. Phillip D. Carter and Peter Rolls; 2015; Blood parasites; Babesiosis; page 1

37. Phillip D. Carter; 2015. Babesiosis sheep and goats; Babesiosis, Circulatory System, Veterinary Manual. *MSD MANUAL Veterinary Manual* 4(4): 4-4. [https://www.msdvetmanual.com/circulatory-system/blood-parasites/babesiosis]

38. PIESMAN J. Emerging tick-borne diseases in temperate climates. *Parasitology Today*, 1987, *3*, 197-199.

39. Piesman, J., and A. Spielman. 1980. Human babesiosis on Nantucket Island: prevalence of *Babesia microti* in ticks. Am. J. Trop. Med. Hyg. 29: 742–746.

40. Piesman, J., and A. Spielman. 1982. *Babesia microti*: infectivity of parasites from ticks for hamsters and white-footed mice. Exp. Parasitol. 53:242–248.

41. Piesman, J., S. J. Karakashian, S. Lewengrub, M. A. Rudzinska, and A. Spielman. 1986. Development of *Babesia microti* sporozoites in adult *Ixodes dammini*. Int. J. Parasitol. 16:381–385.

42. Piesman, J., T. C. Hicks, R. J. Sinsky, and G. Obiri. 1987. Simultaneous transmission of *Borrelia burgdorferi* and *Babesia microti* by individual nymphal *Ixodes dammini* ticks. J. Clin. Microbiol. 25:2012–2013.

43. Rashid A, *et al*; 2010; Prevalence and chemotherapy of babesiosis among Lohi sheep in the Livestock Experiment Station, Qadirabad, Pakistan, and environs; *results and discussion*; volume 16; ISSN 1678-9199; pages 587-59.

44. S. M. Hassan and D. A. Salih, "Bibliography with Ab- stracts, Ticks and Tick-borne Diseases in the Sudan," 1st Edition, Central Laboratory, Ministry of Science and technology, Khartoum, 2009.

45. Saleh, M.A. 2009. Erythrocytic oxidative damage in crossbred cattle naturally infected with Babesia bigemina. Research in Veterinary Science, 86: 43-48. Schalm, O.W., Jain, N.C., Carrol, E.J. 1975. Veterinary Haematology. 3rd Edition Lea and Febiger, Philadephia

46. Schein, E., G. Rehbein, W. P. Voigt, and E. Zweygarth. 1981. *Babesia equi* (Laveran 1901) 1. Development in horses and in lymphocyte culture. Tropenmed. Parasitol. 32:223–227.

47. Sevinc, F., Turgut, K., Sevinc, M., Ekici, O.D., Coskun, A., Koc, Y., Erol, M. and Ica, A. 2007. Therapeutic and prophylactic efficacy of imidocarb dipropionate on experimental Babesia ovis infection of lambs. Vet. Parasitol., 149: 64-71.

48. Spielman, A. 1976. Human babesiosis on Nantucket Island: transmission by nymphal *Ixodes* ticks. Am. J. Trop. Med. Hyg. 25:784–787.

49. Spielman, A., P. Etkind, J. Piesman, T. K. Ruebush II, D. D. Juranek, and M. S. Jacobs. 1981. Reservoir hosts of human babesiosis on Nantucket Island. Am. J. Trop. Med. Hyg. 30:560–565.

50. Stafford, K. C., 3rd. 1991. Effectiveness of carbaryl applications for the control of *Ixodes dammini* (Acari: Ixodidae) nymphs in an endemic residential area. J. Med. Entomol. 28:32–36.

51. Taylor MA, Coop RL, Wall RL. Parasites of cattle: Epidemiology of ostertagiosis in subtropical and temperate countries in the southern hemisphere. In: Veterinary Parasitology. 3rd ed. Oxford: Blackwell Publishing; 2007. p. 57.

52. Taylor MA, Coop RL, Wall RL. Parasites of cattle: Toxocara vitulorum. In: Veterinary Parasitology. 3rd ed. Oxford: Blackwell Publishing; 2007. p. 65–6.

53. Taylor, M.A., Coop, R.L., and Wall, R.L., 2007. Veterinary Parasitology. Third Edn. Blackwell Publishing. PERRY, B. D ., RANDOLPH, T . F., MCDERMOTT, J . J., SONES, K. R. &

THORNTON, P. K. (2002). Investing in animal health research to alleviate poverty. International Livestock Research Institute, Nairobi, Kenya.

54. Wikipedia, (2020). Satellite image of Somaliland, 2017 [Map]. Realsomso. https://commons.wikimedia.org/w/index.php?curid=56173819

55. Telford, S. R., III, A. Gorenflot, P. Brasseur, and A. Spielman. 1993. Babesial infections in humans and wildlife, p. 1–47. *In* J. P. Kreier (ed.), Parasitic protozoa, 2nd ed., vol. 5. Academic Press, San Diego, Calif.

56. Telford, S. R., III, A. Gorenflot, P. Brasseur, and A. Spielman. 1993. Babesial infections in humans and wildlife, p. 1–47. *In* J. P. Kreier (ed.), Parasitic protozoa, 2nd ed., vol. 5. Academic Press, San Diego, Calif.

57. UILENBERG G. Babesiosis, *in*: Encyclopedia of artropod-transmitted infection of man and domesticated animals. Wallingford M.W. (ed.), CABI Publishing, UK, 2001, 122-144.

58. Urquhart GM, J Armour, JL Duncan, AM Dunn, FW Jennings. Veterinary Parasitology. 2nd ed. USA: Blackwell Science Incorporated. 1996; 242- 253.

59. YAKHCHALI M. & HOSSEIN A. Prevalence and ectoparasites fauna of sheep and goats flocks in Urmia suburb, Iran. *Veterinarski Arhiv*, 2006, *76*, 431-442.

ANNEXES

Annex One: Questionnaires

1. Which species of livestock do you keep?

Sheep ☐ Goats ☐ Cattle ☐ Camel ☐ all ☐

2. Have you ever heard about sheep and goat Babesiosis? If yes what do you know about it?

....
....

3. What do you think the causative agent is?

....
....

4. How do you think the disease is transmitted?

....
....

5. What is the local name of camel Babesiosis?

....
....

6. Which types of ticks are present in the area?

....
....

7. Which season is the disease mostly occurs in the area?

Dry season ☐   Wet season ☐

8. Which age group is mostly affected?

Young ☐   Adult ☐

9. Does the disease affect individual animal or herd?

....

10. Which signs do the infected animals manifest?

....
....

11. What are the economic impacts of the Babesiosis in Sheep and Goats?

25

....

....

12. How you treat the Sheep and Goats infected with Babesiosis?

....

....

13. How do you prevent the disease from infecting your Sheep and Goats?

....

....

Annex Two: Field Pictures

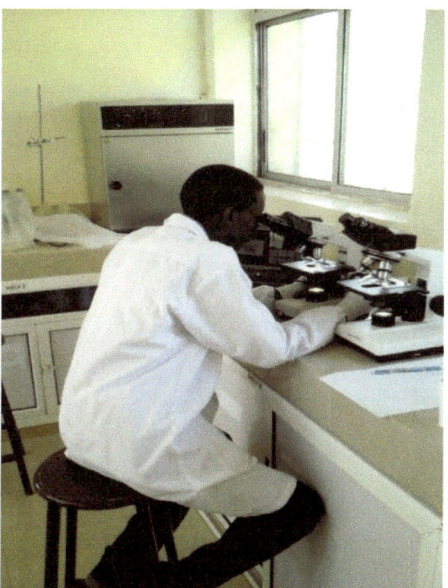

Figure 6: Reading blood smears -own work

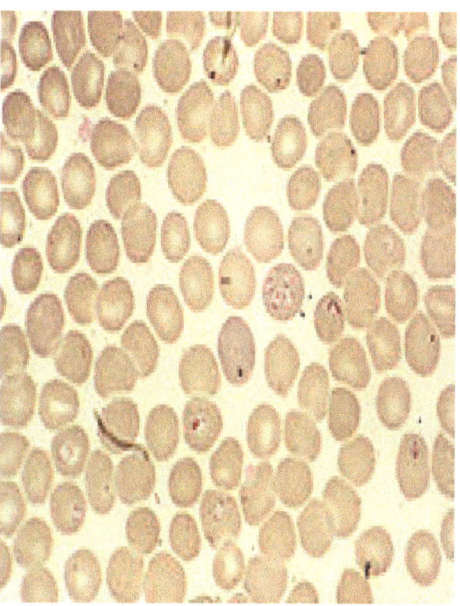

Figure 7: Positive slide of Babesiosis - own work

Annex Three: Map of the Study Area

Figure 8: Map of the study area [Realsomso, 2017]

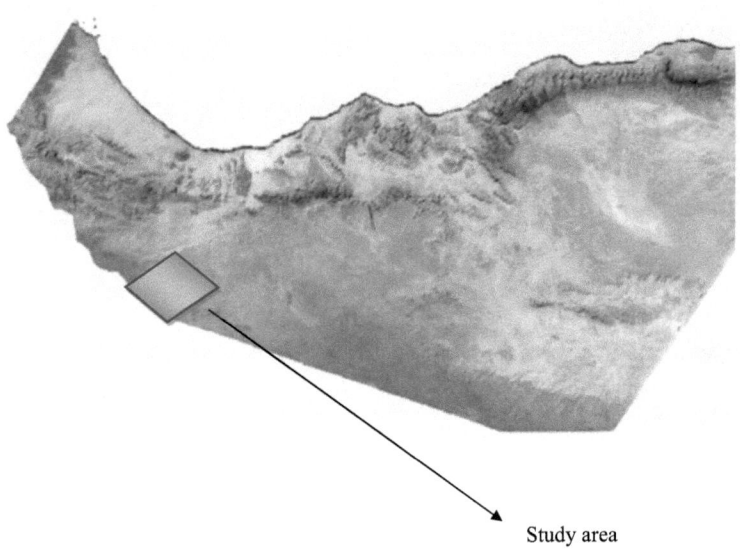

Study area

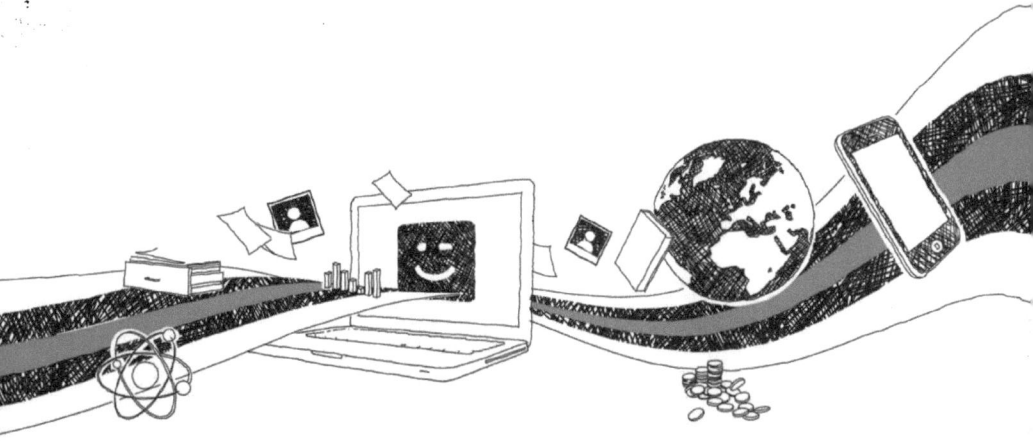
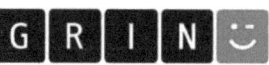